Diabetes and Your Lifestyle
Taking Control of Your Blood Sugar

Daphne Olivier

The Unconventional Dietician

DEDICATION

When I was in dietetic school my dad was diagnosed with diabetes. It was then that I knew I wanted to work with people who were diagnosed with diabetes, as this is a disease of lifestyle. A disease that, while not easy, can be managed by changes to how you live your life. While I would never wish this disease on anyone, I thank my dad for being my inspiration to me to help people live their life to the fullest.

CONTENTS

WHAT HAPPENS WHEN YOU HAVE DIABETES?

Diabetes is a metabolic disorder where the body has difficulty handling the glucose (the fancy medical word for blood sugar) in your blood. The body parts involved in managing blood sugar, include the:

- Liver

- Pancreas

- Each and every body cell, including organ cells, muscle cells, and fat cells

- Various endocrine hormones, most importantly insulin

Glucose, or blood sugar, is found in the blood stream where it is supposed to be. However, blood particles are very particular about how much glucose it is comfortable with in the blood and would rather assist in moving glucose from the blood into every cell of the body where it can be used as its energy source.

There are two ways we get glucose into the blood:

1. *The first is through the foods we eat.* Nearly everything we eat turns into glucose to some degree. Foods with carbohydrates turn to glucose faster and more efficiently. However protein can also be converted if necessary. Fat can be converted into glucose, but it is a more complicated process for the body and it is reserved only for when necessary.

2. *The second way we get glucose in the blood is through the liver.* The liver has the ability to create and hold on to glucose. When your blood glucose begins to drop, a special hormone sends a message to the liver telling it to release its stored glucose. When blood glucose gets back to the normal range a hormone signals the liver telling it to stop releasing glucose. It is a safety mechanism for our body

so we don't have to eat constantly to regulate our glucose. The most common time this occurs is overnight, when we go many hours without eating.

When the levels of blood glucose begin to rise, regardless of whether it came from food or the liver, it signals the pancreas to give little squirts of insulin. When the insulin gets into the blood its job is to attach to a cell receptor site and "open a door" allowing the glucose to move into the cell. Once the glucose is in the cell and no longer in the blood then everyone is happy – the blood has less glucose and the cell is "fed." This is how the dance of managing blood glucose is supposed to work.

When diabetes occurs there are several faults in this system. It usually starts with insulin resistance. This which means that insulin is released from the pancreas but the cell receptors that accept insulin to open the door are resistant to allowing the glucose in. Thus the pancreas must secrete more insulin to allow for the cell to "open the door" for glucose. Suddenly we have a surge of insulin in the blood trying to get the glucose into the cell.

You can think of it like this:

You accidentally get locked out of your house with a young toddler inside. You try to open the door yet you can't. You begin to panic because you need to get inside but all of the doors are locked and not allowing it. You call your neighbors to try to help because you need to get inside. Suddenly there are several neighbors at your house checking for unlocked doors or windows and finally one is open and you can get inside.

When the pancreas releases extra insulin it results in something called *hyperinsulinemia* (extra insulin). The effects of hyperinsulinemia are widespread and very common such as polycystic ovarian disease, high triglycerides, hypertension, damage to endothelial cells leading to coronary artery disease, cardiovascular disease, lethargy, and weight gain. Sometimes the extra squirt of insulin can result in a rapid fall in glucose which can result in blood sugar getting too low, causing a craving for something to eat, usually sweet. This can perpetuate a cycle of high and low blood sugar and can lead to a yo-yo type cycling throughout the day.

MONITORING BLOOD SUGAR

One of the best ways to determine what is going on with your blood sugar at any given time is to test it using a home meter. Monitoring your blood sugar, gives you a snapshot of what is going on at any particular moment. Using this information as an investigative tool provides good clues about the natural rhythm of your blood sugar throughout the day. Some questions you may consider are:

What is my blood sugar when I get up in the morning?

How much does my blood sugar rise after eating meals?

Do certain foods affect my blood sugar more than others?

How does exercise or daily movement affect my blood sugar?

How is my blood sugar affected by stress? Illness? Pain?

All of these questions can be answered by monitoring glucose regularly. There are a few times that are most important times to monitor glucose.

1. First is fasting - in the morning before you've had anything to eat or drink. That fasting blood sugar should ideally be between 70-100mg/dL.
2. The next times are before and after eating a meal. To be specific, monitoring immediately before eating and two hours after you start eating your meal.

Tracking the difference between before you eat and after you eat should be less than 40mg/dl. Anything beyond this indicates that you are not tolerating the carbohydrates with your meal well and the meal should be evaluated.

Example: Before meal 140mg/dL, after meal 160mg/dL

160-140 = 20 Therefore the meal did not have a big effect on glucose because the difference was less than 40

Example: Before meal 90mg/dL, after meal 160mg/Dl

160-90 = 70 therefore the meal did have a big effect on glucose because the difference was more than 40

3. Any time you are active it's helpful to monitor glucose
4. Under any stress whether it's physical stress such as an illness, pain or emotional stress.

Fasting, before anything to eat or drink before all meals	70-100mg/dl
2 hours after you begin your meal	70-140mg/dl

SUPPLEMENTS USEFUL IN GLUCOSE MANAGEMENT

There are many supplements that can be helpful to manage glucose. Some are beneficial because of nutrient deficiencies; however, some are beneficial because of compounds that prove helpful for glucose control.

Alpha Lipoic Acid - Recommended dose: 600mg one to three times per day

- Works well to prevent the onset of diabetes.

- Enhances the uptake of glucose into the cells.

- Helps to improve neuropathy in higher doses (600mg 3xper day).

Berberine - Recommended dose: 500mg 2-3 times per day can be used to lower blood sugar (if gastrointestinal side effects occur decrease dose to 250mg)

- It also works well to decrease cholesterol and triglycerides.

Chromium - Recommended dose: 250-1000mcg per day

- Works well to improve insulin sensitivity and impaired glucose tolerance, specifically in the presence of chromium deficiency.

- Best taken in chromium piccolinate form.

- Chromium should be limited for someone with a history of liver or kidney dysfunction.

Cinnamon - Recommended dose: 1000-6000mg per day

- Best taken as cinnamon cassia

- Works well to improve fasting glucose, triglycerides, total cholesterol, and LDL cholesterol

Coenzyme Q10 (ubiquinol) - Recommended dose: 200mg per day

- Improves insulin secretion and aids in decreasing HgbA1c.

Magnesium (Mg) - Recommended dose: 250-600mg per day

- Works well to improve insulin sensitivity in people who are magnesium deficient.
- The best sources of Mg include Mg citrate or Mg glycinate. Mg citrate also can have a laxative effect and should be started at the lowest dose and incrementally increased. If loose bowels occur decreased the dose.
- Magnesium can also be consumed through taking Epsom salt or Dead Sea salt baths where the magnesium is absorbed through the skin.
- Magnesium oils are also available to spray directly onto the skin for absorption.

Vitamin B12 - Recommended dose: 1000mcg per day

- The use of metformin can cause vitamin B 12 deficiency.
- Best taken in methylcobalamin form.

Vitamin C - Recommended dose: 1000mg daily

- Works well with lowering fasting glucose and after meal glucose levels, especially in conjunction with Metformin.

Vitamin D - Recommended dose: Dependent on vitamin D status, however 2000IU daily is a standard dose

- Supplementation is only recommended when lab tests indicate vitamin D status is less than 60ng per mL where daily amount of vitamin D can be calculated to specifically meet your needs.
- Works well with insulin resistance.

Other nutrients and substances may serve beneficial for glycemic control:

- *Biotin* repletion of deficiency may prove beneficial for insulin sensitivity.

- *Bitter Melon* can be used as a tea or in supplement form to aid with blood sugar control.

- *Inositol* and *Carnitine* can be effective to treat diabetic neuropathy.

- *Glutamine* can help to regulate insulin secretion after meals and improve insulin sensitivity.

- *Zinc* supplementation in light of deficiency can prove to be beneficial.

THE HEALTHY TRINITY

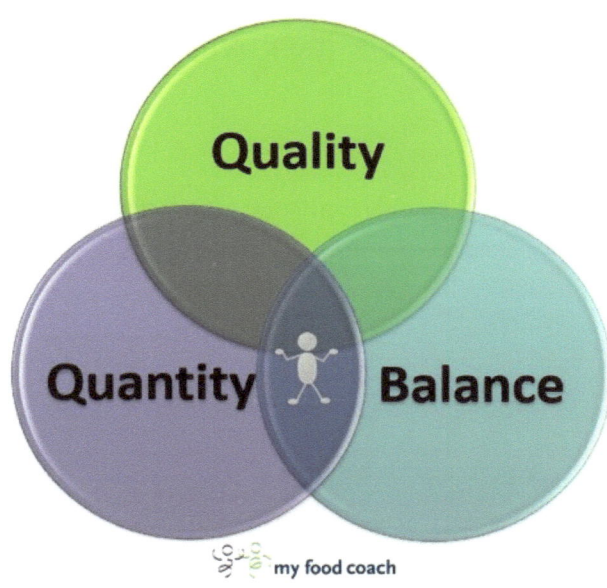

Quality

The *quality* of the foods you choose are just as important at the quantity of the foods you eat.

The *quality* of the thoughts you think make an impact on your ability to be successful.

The *quality* of your relationships and building your support structure will determine your progress.

Quantity

The *quantity* depicts the amount of foods that you consume with each meal.

The *quantity* of stress will negatively affect your health.

The *quantity* of fun you have will prevent food cravings.

Balance

The *balance* of carbohydrates (fiber), protein, and fat.

Balancing your healthy routines of life – meal preparation, monitoring glucose, activity and movement.

Balancing the microbes in your gut to allow for best nutrient absorption and body support.

STOCK THE KITCHEN

Aside from the typical kitchen equipment (fridge,freezer, stove, oven) there are a few additional items that really make food preparation and cooking much easier.

Toaster Oven.

A toaster oven is not appropriate for cooking a meal for the family, but it can be used to heat leftovers (instead of using the microwave), cooking small items, say for only one child, and is much more economical to run than a conventional oven. You can also think of them as a mini-oven which can be used if the conventional oven is already cooking something. They produce significantly less heat which keeps the kitchen cool and you happier. In addition, if you use a toaster oven with a convection feature it can decrease cooking time by as much as 30%. They have a smaller area to clean and some of the high end ones come with a self-cleaning feature. It's just too bad I can't get other things in the house to have a self-cleaning feature.

Slow Cooker

A slow cooker is also known by the brand name Crock Pot®. If you don't have a slow cooker they are worth their weight in gold. If you have one but don't use it, it's time to dust it off and start cooking! There's nothing more satisfying than coming home to a house that smells like the housekeeper has been working hard all day to prepare you a fabulous meal. Also, the cleanup is just one pot.

Food Processor

I love food processors because they are a multi-tasking tool that can be used for bigger projects. There are so many things you can do with a food processor such as making sauces, dips, gravies, pureeing soups, pesto, salsa, soups, grinding spices and nuts, making nut butter, or making bread crumbs. This is a just a few ways to use a food processor, and the only limitation is your imagination.

Immersion or handheld blender

This tool is useful and convenient specifically for small tasks. There's no need to whip out a big blender or processor when you can just submerge your handheld blender into a pot or bowl. These can be used to blend fruit into a smoothie, puree beans into a soup or sauce, emulsify homemade salad dressings, mashing potatoes, making puddings, dips, gravies, and sauces. The list is endless!

In addition here is a list of utensils that are useful.

Set of Good Kitchen Knives

Stock Pot

Sauté pan

Grill Pan

Measuring Spoons

Measuring Cups

Set of Wooden Spoons

Spatula(s)

Parchment Paper

Whisk

Grater

Strainer | Colander

Cutting Boards-*I like a variety of sizes and types*

INGREDIENT ESSENTIALS

When it comes to cooking, there are some basic ingredients you should have on hand that make it easier to pull together a meal, even if you don't have anything planned or if your plan falls through.

PANTRY:

Ingredient	Notes
Arrowroot	Used as a thickening agent to produce a clear gel for sauces & gravies. It thickens at a lower temperature than cornstarch or flour-substitute 2 tsp of arrowroot for 1 tbsp cornstarch, or 1 tsp of arrowroot for 1 tbsp of wheat flour.
Baking Powder	If you are a baker these are essential. If you are not a baker, these are good to have on hand as a leavening agent. Opt for aluminum-free products to prevent heavy metal toxicity.
Baking Soda	
Beans, Dried	Beans have to be prepared to decrease anti-nutrients. Beans must be soaked in warm water with either an acidic (vinegar) or basic (baking soda) medium for at least 24 hours, changing the water at least once during the soaking process before being cooked.
Coconut Oil	Stable oil used for cooking at high temperatures, such as frying (smoking point is 280°F). Coconut oil also offers anti-microbial properties not found in most fats.
Garlic cloves, paste, or powder	Keep whole garlic stored in a dry, low-humid environment with the tops on. Use 1/8 tsp garlic powder to replace 1 garlic clove.
Ghee	A type of clarified butter with the milk solids removed, useful for people who have allergies or sensitivities to milk. This can be used for cooking or frying at high temperatures.

Nuts any variety	All nuts contain the anti-nutrient phytate. Thus soaking nuts for 6 to-18 hours, then dehydrating at very low temperatures eliminates a portion of phytates, allowing your body to easily digest the nuts and to utilize the nutrients. If you frequently eat nuts, the soaking and dehydration is important, however if nuts are not a staple for you it is not as important.
Olive Oil	Cold-pressed extra virgin or virgin olive oil in dark glass-the light causes oxidation & causes rancidity. Olive oil should be used for cold or very low heat preparation.
Onions	Keep whole onions stored in a cool, dark spot in the pantry. However they can be sliced and stored in the freezer for convenience. Conventional onions are on the "clean fifteen" list, meaning they do not hold large amounts of toxins.
Sea Salt	Sea salt naturally has a higher mineral content, which differ depending on where it originates, without the additives found in table salt.
Stevia	If you are looking for a sweetener stevia is a natural sugar replacement. Be sure when you are purchasing stevia is the only ingredient listed.
Tomatoes- whole, sauce, paste	Fresh tomatoes are great for cooking. They can be frozen whole and the skin easily comes off when defrosted. Otherwise, look for tomatoes packaged in glass, as the acidity in the tomatoes can cause the BPA lining of cans to leach into the food.
Vinegar, your favorite variety	Great for use in salad dressings, dips, marinades, sauces, and reductions.

REFRIGERATOR OR FREEZER:

Beef	Grass fed, any cut has significantly more nutrients than conventional beef.
Bell peppers	Keep whole bell peppers stored in the refrigerator if used within 5 days, however they can be sliced and stored in the freezer for convenience.
Broth	Homemade broth, made with bones of any animal is very nourishing to the digestive tract. Do not use broth from a can or box, as they are artificially flavored with MSG.
Butter	Real butter. Don't bother with margarine or "tub butter."
Cheese	Made from raw milk preferably. Otherwise made from milk, cultures, and rennet with minimal added ingredients.
Chicken	Farm fresh, free range, or cage-free chicken to enhance the nutrient content.
Eggs	Farm fresh, free range, or cage free eggs to enhance the nutrient content.
Fruit	Fermented fruit allows the body to utilize the nutrients & enzymes. Otherwise fresh or frozen without added sugar are good options.
Nut butters	The ingredient list should be only the ground nut to make the butter (and maybe salt). Once opened it should be kept in the refrigerator to prevent rancidity. Try a variety of nut or seed butters.
Organ meats	Organ meats are truly a superfood-they are loaded with nutrients that are not found in the same quantities in most foods. Look for organ meats from animals that are pastured for the best nutritional bang for your buck.

Pork	Pastured pork, any cut. Any processed pork that is nitrate-free.
Salsa	Fresh salsa is very versatile and can be used in salads, dips, or preparing meals.
Seafood, wild	Seafood is a great protein source and has nutrients not found in other meat sources.
Vegetables	Otherwise fresh or frozen without added seasoning packs or sauces are good options. Fermented veggies allow the body to utilize the nutrient & enzymes.

PORTION GUIDE

Protein

1 serving = 1 ounce meat = 7g

Meat:
Beef
Buffalo/bison
Chicken
Cornish hen
Duck
Elk
Goat
Goose
Guinea
Lamb
Mutton
Pork
Quail
Rabbit
Turkey
Veal
Venison
Wild game

Organ meats:
Heart
Kidney
Liver
Pate

Seafood
Fish:
Anchovies
Halibut
Herring
Mackerel
Mahi Mahi
Salmon
Sardines, 2 medium
Trout
Tuna

Other Seafood:
Clams
Crabs
Crawfish
Lobster
Mussels
Oysters, 6 medium
Shrimp

Other:
Egg with yolk, 1
Cottage Cheese, ¼ cup

Fats:

Nuts:
Almond/almond butter, 6 whole nuts/1 Tbsp
Brazil nuts, 2 nuts
Cashews/cashew butter, 6 cashews/ 1 Tbsp
Pine nuts, 25 nuts
Pistachios, 25 nuts
Walnuts, 5 halves
Hazelnuts, 5 nuts
Macadamia nuts, 5 nuts
Peanuts | Peanut Butter, 10 nuts, 1 Tbsp
Pecans, 4 halves

Seeds:
Chia seeds, 1Tbsp
Flax seed, freshly ground, 1Tbsp
Hemp seeds, 1 Tbsp
Pumpkin seeds, 1 Tbsp
Sesame seeds, 1 Tbsp
Sunflower seeds/ sunflower seed butter, 1 Tbsp
Tahini, 1 Tbsp

Oils:
1 serving = 1 tsp
Avocado oil
Coconut oil
Flax oil (cold only)
Olive oil(cold pressed, extra virgin)
Palm oil
Sesame oil (cold pressed)

Other Fats:
Avocado, ¼ medium
Bacon fat (from pastured pigs), 1 tsp
Beef tallow, 1 tsp
Butter, 1 tsp
Coconut butter, 1 tsp
Coconut milk, canned, 2 Tbsp
Duck fat, 1 tsp
Ghee, 1 tsp
Lard (from pastured pigs), 1 tsp
Olives, black or green, 8 -10 large

Dairy Fat:
Cheese: 1 serving = 1 ounce
Blue Cheese/Gorgonzola, 1 oz
Brie, 1 oz
Cheddar cheese, 1 oz
Cream cheese, 1 Tbsp
Feta, 1 oz
Gouda, 1 oz
Mozzarella, 1 oz
Parmesan, 1 oz
Pepper jack, 1 oz
Provolone, 1 oz
Ricotta, 1 oz
Swiss, 1 oz

Breakfast	*Lunch*	*Supper*	*Snack*
___Protein	___Protein	___Protein	___Protein
___Fat	___Fat	___Fat	___Fat
___Carbohydrates	___Carbohydrates	___Carbohydrates	___Carbohydrates

Non-Starchy Vegetables (5g/svg)

1 serving = ½ cup cooked or
1 cup raw

Alfalfa sprouts
Artichoke & hearts
Asparagus
Bamboo shoots
Beans (green, Italian, yellow, wax)
Bell peppers
Bok choy
Broccoli
Brussel sprouts
Cabbage
Cauliflower
Celery
Cucumbers
Eggplant
Garlic
Greens (beet, collard, dandelion, mustard, turnip)
Hearts of palm
Jimaca
Kale
Kohlrabi
Leeks
Lettuce (endive, romaine, iceberg)
Mushrooms
Okra
Onions, (chives, shallots)
Pea pods
Peppers (any)
Radishes
Salad greens
Spinach
Summer squash
Swiss chard
Tomatoes
Turnips
Watercress
Zucchini

Fruit
(15g/svg)
Apple (including green), 1 tennis ball size
Applesauce, unsweetened, ½ cup
Apricot, 4 fresh, 8 halves
Banana, ½ large or 1 small
Blackberries, ¾ cup

Fruit Cont'd

Blueberries, ¾ cup
Cantaloupe, 1 cup cubes
Cherries
Dates, 3 medium dried
Figs, 2 medium
Goji berries
Grapes, 17
Grapefruit, ½ fruit
Honeydew melon, 1 cup cubes
Kiwi, 1 large
Mango, ½ small or ½ cup
Nectarine, 1 tennis ball size
Orange, 1 tennis ball size
Peach, 1 tennis ball size
Pears, ½ large
Pineapple, ¾ cup raw, ½ cup canned in water
Plum, 2 small
Pomegranate, ½ cup seeds
Prunes, 3 medium
Raisins, 2 Tbsp
Raspberries, 1 cup
Rhubarb, 2 cups
Strawberries, 1 ¼ cup whole
Watermelon, 1 ¼ cup cubes

Root & Winter Vegetables
(15g/svg)
1 serving = ½ cup
Acorn squash
Beets
Butternut squash
Carrots
Parsnips
Plantains
Pumpkin
Sweet potatoes
White potatoes, ½ cup mashed or 1 small (3 oz)
Winter roots or squash, 1 cup
Yams

Legumes
(15g/svg)
1 serving = ½ cup
Black beans
Black eye peas
Chickpeas (Garbanzo beans)

Legumes Cont'd
Hummus
Lentils
Lima beans
Navy beans
Kidney beans
Peas (dried or split)
Pinto beans
Split peas
White beans

Grains
(15g/svg)
1 serving = ½ cup cooked
Amaranth
Barley
Buckwheat/kasha
Bulgur
Corn
Kamut
Millet
Oats/oatmeal
Polenta
Quinoa
Rice, (white, basmati, brown, jasmine, or wild)
Rye
Sorghum
Spelt
Tapioca
Teff
Whole wheat

(italicized items contain gluten)

Dairy/Dairy Alternative
(12g/svg)
Milk:
Yogurt (plain with live cultures), 6 oz
Cow's milk, 1 cup
Goat's milk, 1 cup

Dairy Alternatives:
Coconut milk, carton, unsweetened 2 cups
Hemp milk, ¾ cup
   *Almond milk, unsweetened
   *Cashew milk, unsweetened

GROCERY LIST

Fresh Fruit
□ Apples
□ Apricots
□ Bananas
□ Blackberries
□ Blueberries
□ Cantaloupe
□ Grapefruit
□ Grapes
□ Guava
□ Honeydew Melon
□ Kiwi
□ Lemons
□ Limes
□ Nectarines
□ Oranges
□ Papaya
□ Peach
□ Plums
□ Raspberries
□ Rhubarb
□ Strawberries
□ Watermelon

Fresh Vegetables
□ Acorn Squash
□ Alfalfa Sprouts
□ Artichoke
□ Asparagus
□ Bamboo Shoots
□ Beans
□ Beet Greens
□ Bok Choy
□ Broccoli
□ Brussel Sprouts
□ Butternut Squash

Fresh Vegetables Cont'd
□ Cabbage
□ Carrots
□ Cauliflower
□ Celery
□ Chives
□ Collard Greens
□ Corn
□ Cucumbers
□ Eggplant
□ Garlic
□ Green Peas
□ Hearts of Palm
□ Jicama
□ Kale
□ Kohlrabi
□ Leeks
□ Lettuce
□ Mushrooms
□ Mustard Greens
□ Okra
□ Onions
□ Peppers
□ Pumpkin
□ Radishes
□ Sea Vegetables
□ Snow Peas
□ Spinach
□ Summer Squash
□ Sweet Potatoes
□ Tomatoes
□ Turnips
□ Turnip Greens
□ Watercress
□ Water Chestnuts
□ Zucchini

Spices & Herbs
□ Basil
□ Black Pepper
□ Cayenne Pepper
□ Cilantro
□ Cinnamon
□ Cumin
□ Garlic
□ Ginger
□ Mint
□ Oregano
□ Paprika
□ Parsley
□ Red Pepper
□ Rosemary
□ Sea Salt
□ Stevia
□ Thyme
□ Turmeric
□ Vanilla Extract

Dairy
□ Butter
□ Buttermilk
□ Half & Half
□ Heavy Cream
□ Kefir
□ Milk
□ Sour Cream
□ Yogurt

Frozen Fruit
□ Frozen Blueberries
□ Frozen Fruit Blend
□ Frozen Peaches
□ Frozen Strawberries

GROCERY LIST

Cheese

- ☐ Blue Cheese
- ☐ Cheddar Cheese
- ☐ Cottage Cheese
- ☐ Cream Cheese
- ☐ Feta Chesse
- ☐ Goat Cheese
- ☐ Gouda
- ☐ Mozzarella
- ☐ Parmesan
- ☐ Provolone
- ☐ Ricotta
- ☐ Swiss

Frozen Vegetables

- ☐ Frozen Okra
- ☐ Frozen Broccoli
- ☐ Frozen Brussel Sprouts
- ☐ Frozen Carrots
- ☐ Frozen Cauliflower
- ☐ Frozen Corn
- ☐ Frozen Green Beans
- ☐ Frozen Greens
- ☐ Frozen Okra
- ☐ Frozen Onions
- ☐ Frozen Potatoes
- ☐ Frozen Seasoning Blend
- ☐ Frozen Spinach
- ☐ Frozen Squash
- ☐ Frozen Veg Medley

Meat

- ☐ Beef
- ☐ Ground Beef
- ☐ Chicken

Refrigerated

- ☐ Eggs

Meat Cont'd

- ☐ Ground Chicken
- ☐ Ground Turkey
- ☐ Heart
- ☐ Kidney
- ☐ Liver
- ☐ Pate
- ☐ Pork
- ☐ Turkey

Seafood

- ☐ Anchovies
- ☐ Clams
- ☐ Crabs
- ☐ Crawfish
- ☐ Herring
- ☐ Lobster
- ☐ Mackerel
- ☐ Mussels
- ☐ Salmon
- ☐ Sardines
- ☐ Scallops
- ☐ Shrimp
- ☐ Tuna
- ☐ Trout

Fats

- ☐ Coconut Oil
- ☐ Olive Oil
- ☐ Palm Oil
- ☐ Pecan Oil
- ☐ Safflower
- ☐ Sesame Oil
- ☐ Walnut

Bathroom Items

- ☐ Antiperspirant
- ☐ Band-Aids
- ☐ Conditioner

Bathroom Items Cont'd

- ☐ Cotton Balls
- ☐ Cotton Swabs
- ☐ Dental Floss
- ☐ Lip Balm
- ☐ Moisturizing Lotion
- ☐ Mouthwash
- ☐ Razors
- ☐ Shampoo
- ☐ Shaving Cream
- ☐ Soap
- ☐ Toilet Paper
- ☐ Toothpaste

Various Groceries

- ☐ Coconut Milk
- ☐ Coffee / Coffee Filters
- ☐ Dried Beans
- ☐ Lemon Juice
- ☐ Lime Juice
- ☐ Nut Butter
- ☐ Oats
- ☐ Olive Oil
- ☐ Olives
- ☐ Rice
- ☐ Tea
- ☐ Tomato Juice
- ☐ Tomato Paste
- ☐ Vinegar

Kitchen Items

- ☐ Freezer Bags
- ☐ Freezer Paper
- ☐ Freezer Tape
- ☐ Napkins
- ☐ Parchment Paper
- ☐ Paper Towels
- ☐ Plastic Wrap
- ☐ Wax Paper

Breakfast Rules

Rule #1 – You *must* eat breakfast

Since breakfast is breaking the fast of the night, it is a vital way to start the day. Numerous studies have linked skipping breakfast to developing obesity, as it greatly impacts your metabolism. In fact, according to the National Weight Control Registry, a volunteer based study of successful long term weight loss, 78% of people who have lost weight and been able to keep it off eat breakfast every day. In adults and kids alike, eating breakfast is also linked to improved cognition, memory, and motor function. So really, weather you eat breakfast or not is non-negotiable.

Rule #2 – Eat breakfast shortly after waking

Not only is eating breakfast uber important, the timing of when you eat also plays a role. Chrono nutrition is the study of your circadian rhythm and metabolism – how time and nutrition play a role in your organs that affect metabolism, your liver, pancreas, fatty tissue, and muscles. While these studies are new, it's suggested that eating within one hour of waking is the ideal time to have your first bites of the day.

Rule #3 – Balance your breakfast

As with all meals, having a balanced breakfast is critical if you want to obtain the benefits of eating breakfast. A balanced breakfast consists of appropriate amounts of protein, healthy fats, and carbohydrates, specifically fiber. While it may take a little planning at first, these can be planned to become second nature when you reach for something in the morning.

Do you want to stop snacking in the evening? Eat a balanced breakfast.

Want to stop cravings in the afternoon? Eat a balanced breakfast.

Want to lose weight? Start with a balanced breakfast.

Balancing Breakfast

Considering items as biscuits, cereal with milk, pancakes, and muffins, traditional breakfast fare is not exactly balanced and resembles desserts rather than a crucial meal to kick-start your day. This means that to build a balanced breakfast you may have to think outside of the box, allowing for some foods that are generally considered more appropriate for lunch or supper.

Remember, a balanced breakfast has 3 components – protein, healthy fat, and fiber.

Breakfast protein

• Pastured, organic eggs – fried, scrambled, poached, boiled

• Homemade chicken, turkey, or pork sausage (see recipe)

• Leftover meats, whole or ground – chicken, beef, pork

• Salmon or other fish

• Full fat cottage cheese

• Full fat Greek yogurt

Healthy breakfast fats

• Butter, preferably grass fed

• Coconut or coconut oil

• Avocado or avocado oil

• Olive oil

• Nuts & seeds or nut butters such as almond butter or sunflower seed butter

• Full fat cheese

Breakfast fiber

- Greens (spinach, collard greens, kale, Swiss chard, etc) or other vegetables

- Root veggies like potatoes, sweet potatoes, carrots, parsnips, or squash

- Chia & flax seeds

- Berries and other fruit in moderation (limit them to about 1/2 – 3/4 cup at a time

- Steel cut oats

BREAKFAST RECIPES

Eggs

Basic Veggie Frittata

Yields 3 servings

3/4 pound veggies-your favorites or leftovers work well

1 large or 2 small leeks

2 Tbsp butter

6 eggs

1/4 cup whole milk

1/4-1/2 tsp **sea salt** or **Himalayan salt**, depending on your taste

black pepper, freshly ground

1/8 tsp nutmeg

1/4 cup cheese, grated-use your favorite such as cheddar, Monterey Jack, or feta (optional)

1. Preheat the oven to 300°F.
2. Slice the leeks into thick rounds. Put them into a bowl with water and mix to get the dirt out.
3. On the stove, melt the butter in an oven safe skillet (cast iron or stainless steel). When hot, remove the leeks from the water, shaking off any excess and put them into the pan.
4. Sauté over medium-high heat until tender.
5. Add your veggies to the pan with about 1 Tbsp water and allow them to cook for 1-3 minutes, covered.
6. Meanwhile, mix together the eggs and milk.

7. Add salt, pepper, and nutmeg.

8. Pour the egg mixture into the skillet over the veggies, then add cheese. Gently press the cheese into the eggs.

9. Let it cook on the stovetop on low heat for 2-3 minutes then transfer to the oven. Bake until the eggs are just set, which can be as little as 5 minutes.

10. Remove from the oven, and allow to cool a few minutes, then slice and serve.

Southwestern Scrambled Eggs

Yields 1 serving

2 eggs

½ cup salsa

¼ cup cheddar cheese (optional)

¼ avocado, sliced

¼ cup onions, diced (optional)

½ jalapeno, seeded & diced (optional)

½ green bell pepper, sliced (optional)

1 Tbsp butter

1. Melt butter in a skillet on medium high heat.

2. If you are using onions, green bell peppers, and jalapenos add to the butter to allow them to cook until your desired tenderness.

3. Beat eggs & salsa in a bowl and then pour into the hot skillet with the onion mixture. Reduce heat to medium and cover skillet.

4. After 3-4 minutes scrape and lift the edges of the eggs and begin to "scramble" the eggs mixture in the skillet allowing the uncooked portion to cook.

5. When the eggs are cooked, remove from the skillet and add cheese and avocado.

Banana Egg "Pancakes"

Yields 2 servings

3 eggs

1 banana

1 tsp cinnamon

1 pinch sea salt or Himalayan salt

1 tsp butter

1. Preheat skillet over medium heat while preparing food.
2. Place eggs, banana, cinnamon and salt in blender and blend until smooth. (You don't want any chunks of banana floating around)
3. Melt butter in skillet and add egg mixture.
4. Cook until eggs begin to set and flip. Cook until fully set and enjoy with bacon, sausage, or sweet potato hash browns.

Zucchini Patties

Yields 5 servings

2 medium zucchini

1 Tbsp sea salt or Himalayan salt

½ cup cheese, your favorite, but I've used mozzarella, parmesan, and feta

2 eggs

½ tsp thyme

1-2 Tbsp butter

1. Wash the zucchini well, and then grate using a food grater.
2. Put the grated zucchini in a mixing bowl, sprinkle 1 Tbsp salt on top of zucchini and cover with water. Allow it to sit for 1 hour (the salt pulls the fluid out of the zucchini so it holds better).

3. Drain the zucchini then use a cotton towel to squeeze as much water as possible out of the zucchini. If the zucchini still has water in it the patties will become "runny" (although it will not affect the taste, it will be hard to keep the patties together).

4. Once the water has been squeezed out of the zucchini, mix in a bowl with eggs, cheese, and thyme.

5. Form the zucchini into small patties. Melt butter in a skillet on low-medium. Place the zucchini in the skillet and allow them to cook slowly, making sure they are completely cooked on one side before attempting to flip.

6. Flip patties to ensure they are well-cooked on both sides.

Dairy

Cottage Cheese (full fat) with fruit, nuts/seeds (almond slivers, walnuts, pecans, cashews, sunflower, pumpkin, or chia seeds)

Greek yogurt, full fat, plain with fruit and nuts/seeds

Other

Breakfast Sausage

Yields 8 patties

1 pound ground meat-pork, chicken, beef, turkey or a mix

1 tsp salt

1 tsp sage

1 tsp basil or marjoram

1 tsp white pepper

1 tsp garlic powder

1 tsp onion powder

½ cup water

1 tbsp coconut oil, or other frying fat

1. Put all ingredients in a mixing bowl. Wet hands, then mix all ingredients together.

2. Melt the coconut oil or fat in a skillet on medium–high heat.

3. Divide the ground meat into small balls a little larger than a golf ball, then flatten and pan fry in the skillet.

4. Allow to fry on one side for 3-5 minutes, then flip and allow them to fry on the other side.

Sweet Potato Niblets

Yields 4-6 servings depending on size of potatoes

2 large sweet potatoes, peeled & cubed

2 tbsp coconut oil

To Taste: Sea salt or Himalayan salt

1. Preheat oven to 425ºF.

2. Place cubed sweet potatoes & coconut oil into a gallon sized zip top bag. Shake and agitate until the sweet potatoes are lightly covered with coconut oil.

3. Pour oil-covered sweet potatoes into a single layer on a parchment paper lined cookie sheet (parchment paper makes cleaning EASY) and bake for 20 minutes. Pull sweet potatoes out of oven, sprinkle with sea salt and flip the potatoes. Bake for an additional 15-20 minutes.

Fruit & Seed Granola

Yields 8-½ cup servings

1 cup pumpkin seeds

1 cup sunflower seeds

1 cup coconut flakes, unsweetened

1/4 cup honey, warmed

Pinch: Sea salt or Himalayan salt

1/2 tbsp vanilla extract

2 tsp cinnamon

1 cup dried fruit, any variety, cut up

1. Preheat oven to 350°F. Grease a large pan or line with parchment paper.

2. Mix all ingredients except dried fruit and toss well.

3. Spread on baking sheet and bake until golden brown, approximately 20 minutes, stirring every 5 minutes.

4. Remove from the oven and stir in dried fruit. Continue to stir every few minutes during the cooling process.

5. Keep in an airtight container at room temperature.

Apple or Banana with Nut Butter Smear

Slice the fruit into 8 pieces (the banana can be cut into fourths, then in half making a flat side) and smear with sunflower seed butter, almond butter, cashew butter, or any other nut butter you enjoy.

Fruit & Nut Salad

Yields 2 servings

1/2 apple, cored and diced

2-3 strawberries, sliced

1/4 cup blueberries

1/8 cup coconut, shredded & unsweetened

1/4 cup walnuts or pecans, chopped

1/2 tsp cinnamon (optional)

1. Place all fruit into a bowl.

2. *Sprinkle with coconut, nuts, and cinnamon (optional).*

BUILD YOUR OWN SMOOTHIE

Liquid 1 Serving size: 6-8 oz.	Vegetable 1 Serving size: 1 cup	Fat 1 Serving size: 1 tsp	Protein 1 Serving size: 7g	Fruit (optional) 1 Serving size: 1 piece
Cow or Goat's milk	Spinach	Coconut oil	Collagen powder	Banana
Almond milk	Kale	Canned coconut milk	Whey protein Powder	Strawberries
Coconut milk		Nuts (almonds, cashews, walnuts)	Egg white Protein Powder	Blueberries
Plain yogurt				Raspberries
Kefir		Nut butters (almond, peanut, or sunflower seed butter)	Rice Protein Powder	Blackberries
Water			Pea Protein Powder	Mangoes
		Seeds (chia seeds, pumpkin seeds, sunflower seeds)	Vegetable Protein Powder	
		Avocado		*frozen makes it smooth and creamy

1. In the blender, add 6-8 ounces of the liquid of your choice per serving.
2. Add frozen fruit, equivalent to 1 piece of fruit per serving, and veggie, about 1 cup.
3. Add your choice of fat and protein powder, then blend all together and serve.

BUILD YOUR OWN MEAL

CREATE YOUR OWN SALAD **Choose Your Greens- Unlimited:**	*Choose Your Protein-4-6 ounces per adult*	**Create Your Own Salad Dressing-**
Kale (baby, dinosaur, curly) Spinach Bok choy Mustard greens Arugula Cabbage Romaine lettuce	Chicken Turkey Beef Pork Salmon Sardines	3 parts oil : 1 part vinegar *Choose Your Oil* Extra- virgin olive oil Avocado oil *Flax oil*
Choose Your Vegetables- any combination: Cucumber Carrots Broccoli Cauliflower Asparagus Zucchini Yellow squash Roasted or grated fresh Beets Onion Celery	*Choose Your Sweetness (optional & minimal)* Apples Pears Oranges Dried unsweetened Cranberries Dried unsweetened cherries Unsweetened coconut flakes	*Choose Your Vinegar* Apple cider vinegar Balsamic vinegar *Choose Your Juice (Optional)* Lemon juice Lime juice Orange juice
	Top with Herbs/Spices(optional) Cilantro Mint Parsley Basil Freshly grated ginger root	*Choose Your Seasoning* Sea salt Ground black pepper Minced garlic Minced onion or shallot Fresh herbs: basil, cilantro, mint, parsley Spices: cinnamon, turmeric

HOW TO BUILD A MEAL

Meal planning is a game that is limited only by your imagination. It takes time and preparation, but in the end you will win satisfaction and enthusiasm fr om yourself and your family. To start, celebrate where you are in the process right now. Just that fact that you want to make changes to your current situation is a good place to start. Next, you will make certain that your kitchen is well stocked. That means everything from preparation materials such as canning jars and zip top bags, to having a stocked pantry with spices and herbs for flavoring, to having space in the freezer. Then you can get started with planning meals.

Start by asking each person what their favorite meals are and use that as a springboard to get your meal planning strategies going. If you are like me, each person has their own idea of what the perfect meal is and it can change every time you ask. One person likes one thing and the other likes something opposite. That's okay, we can (almost always) please everyone.

This will become your toolbox for planning meals. This "toolbox" will have whatever you need in it to inspire you, but I recommend the recipe or a reminder of the meal if you can make it without a recipe. For instance, I don't need a recipe for tacos, but it is such an easy meal to forget if it's not written down somewhere. This toolbox can even go as far as writing down the food list along with it. That makes it easier to quickly review and learn what you have on hand and what you need.

Create a schedule and stick to it. Be realistic about your planning schedule. If you know you will be getting home late one night plan for it. Or if the day starts early, make sure you have a quick meal that you can grab and go. Plan meals for several days at one time to avoid monotony and duplication as well as saving time and money.

Make a food list and use it. This list should always be available to mark on, but specifically used throughout the planning process. When you know what the meals will be, you review the recipe(s) for ingredients and write down what you need. This will assure you don't get home from food shopping without the one thing that is needed to "make the recipe."

Display your menu where you and the rest of the family can see it. This will let everyone know what to expect and can serve as a reminder that you need to thaw meat. It keeps you accountable to the meal planning process you have spent time creating.

Introduce new foods occasionally and take a family vote. Was the meal worth making again? If so, jot down any ideas or reminders needed to perfect the meal and add it into rotation.

Always, always, always, keep a few back up meals ready in the freezer. Since life can sometimes be unpredictable, this will keep you prepared for the unexpected.

CREATE YOUR OWN MEAL

Choose Your Protein:
4-6 ounces per adult
Prepared baked, grilled, sautéed, roasted, or slow cooked:
Beef
Lamb
Pork
Chicken
Turkey
Duck
Fish
Shellfish
Wild Game

Choose Your Vegetable:
Unlimited
Leafy Greens: *Kale, Spinach, Collards, etc.*
Green veggies: *Asparagus Broccoli, etc.*
Colorful veggies: *Red Cabbage, Carrots, Beets, etc.*

Alfalfa sprouts
Artichoke
Asparagus
Beans: *Green, Italian, Yellow, Wax*
Beets
Bell Peppers
Bok Choy
Broccoli
Brussel Sprouts
Cabbage
Carrots
Cauliflower
Celery
Cucumbers
Eggplant
Greens: *Beet, Collard, Dandelion, Mustard, Turnip*
Jicama
Kale
Kohlrabi
Lettuce: *Endive, Romaine, Iceberg*
Mushrooms
Okra

Onions, Leeks, Chives
Pea pods
Peppers: *any*
Radishes
Sauerkraut
Spinach
Summer Squash
Swiss Chard
Tomatoes
Turnips
Zucchini

Choose Your Starch:
½-1 cup
Sweet potatoes
Butternut squash
Acorn squash
Spaghetti squash

Choose Your Fat
Coconut oil
Olive oil
Avocado
Olives

MEAL PLANNING RECIPES

Creamy Sweet Potato Soup

1 onion, chopped

2 tbsp **coconut oil**, butter, or other nutrient dense cooking fat

2 tsp ground **cumin**

32 oz. chicken broth

3-4 sweet potatoes, peeled and cubed

1 cup kefir (unsweetened) or plain yogurt

2 tbsp parsley or cilantro

1. Add butter and chopped onion to a 3 quart saucepan on medium-high heat. Saute until the onions are translucent, and then add cumin.
2. Add the chicken broth and cubed sweet potatoes and bring to a boil. Reduce the heat and simmer the soup for 20-25 minutes, until the sweet potatoes are tender.
3. Add kefir or plain yogurt, then using a hand blender; blend the ingredients together to make a puree.
4. Add parsley or cilantro and serve hot.

Butternut Squash Soup

1 onion, chopped

1 Tbsp coconut oil, butter, or other cooking fat

1 red apple, peeled and chopped

2 cups chicken broth

1/3 cup coconut milk, canned

2 cups butternut squash, cubed

1 tsp cumin

1 tsp good quality sea salt or Himalayan salt

1. On medium heat melt the coconut oil or other fat in a stock pot, then add onion. Allow them to cook until they get soft and translucent.

2. Add apples and allow them to cook until they get soft. Add cumin and stir well.

3. Add chicken broth, butternut squash and salt and cover. Allow it to cook until the butternut squash cooks and softens, about 20 minutes.

4. Puree with a stick of butter until smooth, then add coconut milk and stir before serving.

Shrimp, Okra, and Tomato Stew

2 Tbsp refined coconut oil

1 onion, chopped

2 pounds small okra, washed and sliced into 1/2 inch pieces

4 medium ripe tomatoes (1 1/2 pounds), cored, peeled, seeded, and chopped

1/2 cup seafood stock or water

1 small-medium jalapeno, stemmed, seeded, and minced (optional)

1/2 tsp high quality sea salt

1 bay leaf

2 Tbsp fresh parsley, minced

2 pounds shrimp, peeled and deveined

1. Heat oil in a large pot. Add onion and jalapeno and sauté over medium heat until the onion is golden, about 5 minutes.

2. Add the okra and sauté until it starts to soften, about 5 minutes.

3. Add the tomatoes, water, bay leaf, and salt. Bring to a boil, then reduce heat, cover, and simmer for about 15 minutes, until the okra is tender.

4. Remove the cover, raise the heat.

5. Add the shrimp and cook until the liquid thickens, about 5 minutes. You want this dish to be juicy, so simmer until liquid is no longer watery.

6. Stir in parsley and serve when thickened to your desired consistency.

Chicken Tandoori

1 teaspoon curry powder

1 teaspoon turmeric

1 teaspoon paprika

1 teaspoon garlic powder

½ teaspoon white pepper

1 teaspoon sea salt or Himalayan salt

2 cups (1 can) canned coconut milk

1 sweet potato, peeled and diced

1 whole cut up chicken or 4 leg quarters, bone in

1. Add all ingredients in a Dutch oven and cook on stove top on medium low for 35-45 minutes or until no pink runs from the chicken when cut.

2. OR you can add all ingredients to a crock pot and cook on low heat for 4-6 hours.

3. Allow to sit for 10 minutes before serving.

4. Serve warm as a stew.

Chicken & Spinach Meatballs

1 Onion, chopped

2 cups fresh spinach, loosely packed

2 cloves garlic

1 1/2 tsp Herbamare or your favorite salted seasoning blend

1 1/2 lb boneless, skinless chicken thigh or breast, cut into 2" squares

1 tbsp Refined coconut oil or other cooking fat

1. Place the spinach, onion, garlic, and seasoning in a high powered blender or food processor. Pulse a few times.

2. Add the chicken and process until the chicken is ground, but do not let it get too runny.

3. With wet hands, form the mixture into meatballs or patties, whichever you prefer and set on a plate.

4. Heat the coconut oil over medium heat in a skillet and add the meatballs, allowing them to cook for 4-5 minutes, then turn them and allow to cook a little longer, until no longer pink.

Eggplant Stuffed Bell Pepper Boats

¾-1 cup cooked brown rice

4 bell peppers, red, yellow, or green

1 medium onion, diced

2 garlic cloves, minced

1 lb grass fed ground beef

1 eggplant

1 tbsp cooking fat, rendered lard or butter

1 tsp Italian seasoning

1 teaspoon sea salt or Himalayan salt

Freshly ground black peppercorns

Pinch cayenne pepper

Paprika

1. If you haven't already made the rice, prepare the rice following the package instructions.

2. Cut the tops off of the bell peppers. Remove and discard the stem and seeds.

3. Bring a pot of water to a boil and, then place bell peppers cut side up and allow to boil for 6-8 minutes and then remove from the water. Cut them into 4 pieces, or "boats."

4. While the bell peppers are boiling, place the cooking fat in a skillet, then add the onion and garlic. Allow them to cook until the onion is translucent and they are aromatic. Add the ground beef, Italian seasoning, black and cayenne pepper.

5. While cooking, peel and dice the eggplant into dice-sized pieces and then add it to the ground beef mixture.

6. When the ground beef and eggplant are cooked, stir in the rice.

7. In a glass dish, place the bell pepper boats cut size up. Gently fill the boats with the ground beef, mixture.

8. Sprinkle the tops generously with paprika.

9. Place on middle rack and cook for 20-30 minutes and then serve warm.

Teriyaki Chicken

2 lbs chicken, either drumsticks or thighs

1/2 cup soy sauce or coconut aminos *if soy-free*

1/2 cup rice vinegar

1/4 cup honey

1/2 tsp ginger, dried

2 garlic cloves, minced

1. Wash off chicken and place in a small casserole dish to marinate.
2. Combine the rest of the ingredients and stir well.
3. Pour over the meat, cover, and place in the fridge and allow to marinate for a few hours or up to overnight.
4. Preheat oven to 425°F. Place chicken with sauce in oven and cook for 25-30 minutes, or until cooked through.
5. To test, pierce one with a knife all the way to the bone, if it's done the juices will run clear, it not, it will contain a little bit of blood.

Coconut Curry Baked Chicken

4 lbs chicken pieces, legs, wings, thigh

3/4 cup coconut Milk

2 tbsp tamari or coconut aminos

2 tbsp garlic, minced

2 tbsp lime juice

1 tsp turmeric, ground

1 tsp curry powder

1. Place the chicken in a large glass dish just big enough to hold all the pieces.

2. Whisk together the remaining ingredients in a large bowl. Pour the marinade over the chicken and turn to coat. Cover the dish with plastic wrap or aluminum foil and refrigerate. Allow to marinate for 2-8 hours.

3. Preheat the oven to 350°F.

4. Drain the chicken and discard the marinade.

5. Bake chicken for 45 minutes or until the juices run clear when pierced with a fork and internal temperature reaches 165°F.

Shrimp & Veggie Stir-Fry

1 lb shrimp, fresh or thawed

½-1 onion, chopped

1 bell pepper, seeded and chopped *feel free to use red or yellow bell peppers*

2-4 garlic cloves, minced

3 whole carrots, grated

1 cup broccoli, chopped

¼ cup tamari or coconut aminos

2 tsp coconut oil, butter, or other nutrient dense cooking fat

¼ tsp cayenne pepper or black pepper

To taste - sea salt or Himalayan salt

1. Heat butter or coconut oil in a wok or skillet and add shrimp and pepper. Cook 3-4 minutes until pink then set aside.

2. Add onions, garlic, peppers, broccoli, and carrots. Add soy sauce and cook until vegetables are desired tenderness. Add shrimp back to pan and add salt to taste.

3. Toss well and serve.

Spaghetti Squash Pizza Pie

1 spaghetti squash

1 onion, diced

1 tbsp coconut oil

8 oz (1/2 lb) ground beef, preferably grass fed

1½ cup pizza sauce

2 tsp garlic powder

2 tsp paprika

2 tsp parsley

2 tsp Italian seasoning

½ tsp sea salt or himalayan salt

1 tsp white pepper

¾ cup parmesan cheese

3 Eggs

1. Preheat oven to 400 degrees F.
2. Cut spaghetti squash in half lengthwise.
3. Place cut side down in a baking dish with ½" water, cover and put in oven to steam for 30 minutes or until you can poke through the squash with a fork.
4. While squash is steaming, put onion and coconut oil in a sauté pan over medium heat and allow the onion to cook until translucent, about 5 minutes.
5. Add ground beef and cook until the beef is no longer pink, then add pizza sauce, garlic powder, paprika, Italian parsley, Italian seasoning, salt, and pepper.
6. Once squash has steamed, allow the squash to cool, then "thread" the squash into an 8x8 baking dish.

7. Mix the spaghetti squash, beef mixture, and Parmesan cheese in the baking dish.

8. Add the whisked eggs and mix well.

9. Place in the oven uncovered and bake for 40 minutes or until the top of the pie forms a slight crust.

Real Food Starters are the fast and easy ways to combine various foods to create snacks

Fruits and veggies
Nuts and seeds or nut/seed butters
Cheese slices, chunks, rounds, sticks
Olives
Avocado
Sardines

Greek yogurt, full fat, plain OR cottage cheese
  + fruit-berries, mangoes, pineapples, bananas
  + nuts or seeds
	Salmon patties
	Salmon lettuce wraps
	Salmon salad
	Tuna salad

Veggies or plantain chips
  + hummus OR
    Guacamole OR
    Salsa
	Turkey lettuce wraps
	Chicken lettuce wraps
	Chicken salad

Chia pod/chia pudding	Homemade gelatin gummies or Jell-O™
Epic bars Tanka bars Beef jerky *without MSG*	Lara bars Kind bars

ABOUT THE AUTHOR

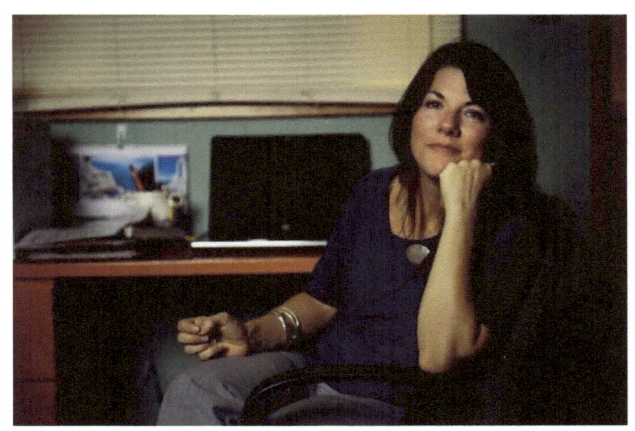

Daphne Oliver is a food passionista, farm girl wanna-be, and registered, yet unconventional dietitian. She graduated Magna Cum Laude from the University of Louisiana; completed her dietetic internship through the VA system in Tampa, Florida; then went on to complete a mentorship with Dr. Liz Lipski, a board member for the Institute of Functional Medicine. She has been a Certified Diabetes Educator since 2009 and is the founder of My Food Coach, her private nutrition practice. She works with people with varying degrees of metabolic disorders including insulin resistance, metabolic syndrome, prediabetes, types 1 and 2 diabetes, and polycystic ovarian syndrome. In her practice she is devoted to providing education, empowerment, and strategies needed to facilitate change to nourish the body and support a healthy lifestyle. Her blog was voted in the Top 100 Blogs by the Psychology of Eating in 2015.

www.ingramcontent.com/pod-product-compliance
Lightning Source LLC
Chambersburg PA
CBHW041513280526
45792CB00004B/1235